Aloe Vera

Six thousand years of medicinal history can't be wrong.

What the pharmaceutical industry doesn't want you to know yet was common knowledge during Cleopatra's time.

Peter Carl Simons

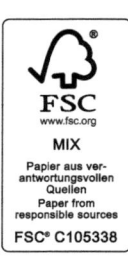

Bibliografische Information der Deutschen Nationalbibliothek:

Die Deutsche Nationalbibliothek verzeichnet diese Publikation in der Deutschen Nationalbibliografie; detaillierte bibliografische Daten sind im Internet über http://dnb.dnb.de abrufbar.

Herstellung und Verlag: BoD –
Books on Demand, Norderstedt

ISBN: 978-3-7526-2657-5

Introduction

By using this book, you accept this disclaimer in full.

No advice

The book contains information. The information is not advice and should not be treated as such.

No representations or warranties

To the maximum extent permitted by applicable law and subject to section below, we exclude all representations, warranties, undertakings and guarantees relating to the book.

Without prejudice to the generality of the foregoing paragraph, we do not represent, warrant, undertake or guarantee:

- that the information in the book is correct, accurate, complete or non-misleading.

- that the use of the guidance in the book will lead to any particular outcome or result.

Limitations and exclusions of liability

The limitations and exclusions of liability set out in this section and elsewhere in this disclaimer: are subject to section 6 below; and govern all liabilities arising under the disclaimer or in relation to the book, including liabilities arising in contract, in tort (including negligence) and for breach of statutory duty.

We will not be liable to you in respect of any losses arising out of any event or events beyond our reasonable control.

We will not be liable to you in respect of any business losses, including without limitation loss of or damage to profits, income, revenue, use, production, anticipated savings, business, contracts, commercial opportunities or goodwill.

We will not be liable to you in respect of any loss or corruption of any data, database or software.

We will not be liable to you in respect of any special, indirect or consequential loss or damage.

Exceptions

Nothing in this disclaimer shall: limit or exclude our liability for death or personal injury resulting from negligence; limit or exclude our liability for fraud or fraudulent misrepresentation; limit any of our liabilities in any way that is not permitted under applicable law; or exclude any of our liabilities that may not be excluded under applicable law.

Severability

If a section of this disclaimer is determined by any court or other competent authority to be unlawful and/or unenforceable, the other sections of this disclaimer continue in effect.

If any unlawful and/or unenforceable section would be lawful or enforceable if part of it were deleted, that part will be deemed to be deleted, and the rest of the section will continue in effect.

Law and jurisdiction

This disclaimer will be governed by and construed in accordance with Swiss law, and any disputes relating to this disclaimer will be subject to the exclusive jurisdiction of the courts of Switzerland.

Contents

Preface

Dear Readers,

Before you continue, please be aware, that all statements and assertions in this book are based on personal experiences and six thousand-year-old insights, as well as knowledge of natural medicine.

It is, therefore, important to recognize that these statements and assertions found here are not based on scientific facts nor are they a recommendation to copy or a promise of healing.

If we're honest, no one within medicine can make that statement. There is no one medicine or drug, regardless of how long it was tested, that works successfully 100% of the time.

All products derived from aloe vera are excluded from patentability, therefore unable to generate huge profits for any one industry or entity. Anyone can grow aloe vera on his or her windowsill. A few hundred years ago, the aloe vera plant was part of the common man's apothecary, cultivated by many. A period followed where the cultivation of the aloe vera plant receded. Today, the plant has resurfaced, grown in popularity and has been recognized for its healing properties, to be used in many different capacities.

Commercial and corporate interest in the development and research of the therapeutic properties of aloe vera is second to none.

Aloe vera contains over 160 components, most of which have a positive effect on our health and well-being. Thousands of years of usage can be attributed to successful cures. Even without the guarantee of a cure it makes sense, in our opinion, to take a closer look, while simultaneously examining our own state of well-being and health. Please consult a medical professional before you try anything.

We wish you a good read and good health!

Peter Carl Simon

The Plant

There are over three hundred scientifically researched aloe vera plants. The aloe vera barbadensis (Miller) is of particular interest. It belongs to the liliaceae or lily family and therefore related to the onion, garlic and asparagus.

Aloe vera is one of the oldest plants with healing properties known to man and has been in use for over six thousand years. The plant grows in regions with a hot, dry summer and mild winters, such as Latin and South America.

Even though the plant itself has a high water content, and is a source for moisture, it needs little water to flourish. The aloe vera stands up to one and a half meters tall with blossoms up to two meters surviving long dry spells and loves intense sunshine.

The plant ripens over a period of three years in sunny, arid regions. In our regions (Central Europe) it takes up to five years. That is the duration the plant needs for all of its 160 beneficial elements to develop and ripen.

A plant with History

The first recordings on the medicinal properties and applications of aloe vera can be found on a shard of earthenware in cuneiform script. This fragment dates back to 4200 BC, found in Babylonia, and is seen as one of the first sources of medicinal prescriptions ever. In old Babylon and Assyria, aloe vera was mixed with absinthe to help with constipation.

Other cultures and societies knew about and used the properties of aloe vera. In the Ebers[1] Papyrus, the use of aloe vera is described in conjunction with healing properties for kidney ailments and the digestive tract. The gel, won from the plant, was also

---

[1] Egyptian Writing from the 18th dynasty - circa 1500 BC

mentioned and used for its cosmetic properties. Women applied the gel topically to re-
tain their youthful skin. Pharaohs put aloe
vera gel in a daily drink in the belief to pro-
long life[2]. Aloe Vera was also used for em-
balming and the mummification process.

---

[2] reason for the name 'immortal plant'

In ancient times, aloe vera was planted in and around the great pyramids[3], seen as a symbolic escort for the rulers to the afterlife. Usage of the plant in Egypt was widespread, proven by sprawling aloe vera plantations that existed during antiquity.

Hippocrates[4] described in his writings the beneficial properties of aloe vera when dealing with ulcers and gastrointestinal disorders. The application of aloe vera was recommended for open wounds, hemorrhoids, abscesses and eye infections by Pedanius Dioscorides[5]. Galen[6] reported on the blood-purifying properties.

---

[3] 3000 BC

[4] Hippocrates of Kos, circa 460-370 BC

[5] The most famous pharmacologist of Antiquity, circa 100 AC - author of »De Materia Medica«.

[6] Galenos of Pergamon, Greek physician and

Much more evidence from the Orient, Africa, Japan and China proves aloe vera has been a source of healing since information of this type has been recorded. Evidence from the New World - Native Americans, the Mayan culture, as well sources from India, tell us aloe vera has been an ingredient used within Ayurveda[7]. One can guess at the importance of aloe vera in Occidental medicine when we see it referred to as 'doctor aloe' by the school of Salerno[8].

---

anatomist, circa 100 AC

[7] It is assumed that ayurveda is over 5000 years old..

[8] an excerpt from Wikipedia:

"The monastery of Monte Cassino hosted a hospital in Salerno for sick friars. Ships docked in Salerno, to have their patients taken care of. One of the first medical schools in Europe was developed out of a group of healers - the civitas salernitatis. Under Archbishop Alfanus and with help from Constantine Africanus, a Christian-

Arabic medical doctor from Tunisia, who translated greek-arabic medical texts into latin, the school flourished and reached its prime between the 10th and 13th century. The school was sponsored by Roger II. and the Holy Roman Emperor Friedrich II..

Comprehensive pharmacology was solidified with the books Liber Graduum, Antidotarium Nicolai and Circa instans. With this knowledge, the apothecaries profession became independent and was separated from the medical profession and was decreed so by law - known as the edict of Salerno - by Friedrich II.

Anatomical studies done on pigs increased medical knowledge with the assumption, that there are parallels between the human body and that of the pig. The school's recipe for success was based on the harmonious blend between the different cultures in regards to medicinal science: the Greek, the Arabic, Western European and the Jewish cultures. Women were accepted into the study program as well as being allowed to teach."

Aloe vera was recommended to cure/heal oozing wounds, eye discharge, earaches, digestive disorders, exhaustion, liver problems and hair loss. Paracelsus[9], a member of the school of Salerno, encountered aloe vera during his studies there. He used the 'golden liquid' to treat burns and illness caused by poison.

Countless other well-known and respected researchers, physicians and pharmacologists have written about the properties of aloe vera. But since we are more interested in the effects of the plant, we will leave the historical view to existing sources and content.

---

[9] Philippus Theophrastus Aureolus Bombastus of Hohenheim, 1493 (Egg, Schwyz, Switzerland) - 1541 (Salzburg, Austria)

Also in modern history, many researchers, medical practitioners and other professionals have recorded their findings on the healing properties of aloe vera. It is unfortunate that these results have been largely ignored. I would, however, like to direct your attention to a wonderful book by Prof. Hademar Bankhofer[10], who offers a cogent and comprehensive overview on aloe vera.

---

[10] See literary list.

Over 160 Proven Properties

A plant with over 160 substantiated substances finds usage in the most diverse areas, one reason why the Egyptians called it the immortal plant. They established that the usage of this plant achieved positive results for many maladies.

In our modern world, we tend to inflict upon our bodies daily stress, unhealthy meals, alcohol, nicotine, polluted air and lack of exercise, to then try and counterbalance the negative effects by popping vitamins. It should be common sense, that these habits are not beneficial nor of lasting success. It is the same as if you would bash the exterior of a car all day with all the tools at your disposal and then try and fill all the holes, bruises and dents with a filler. It may conceal the problems short term, to keep up appearances, but the longevity of the car will suffer dramatically.

Having said that, we have no control over some of these negative influences we are subjected to (air pollution for example) which is why we turn to the aloe vera barbadensis (Miller) for its amazing properties, that can be taken to counteract these influences. The plant can supply the body with important vital substances needed to support the body in self-regeneration. Let's take a closer look at some these properties.

Bioflavonoids - Anti-bacterial, Anti-inflammatory

The secondary plant substances of aloe vera, or bioflavonoids, belong to the plant's most important properties. Aloe vera contains a multitude of elements from this group, with differentiating degrees of healing. The following bioflavonoids are in the aloe vera:

- Lignins are easily absorbed into the skin for an anti-inflammatory effect

- Saponaria have active anti-bacterial effects, stemming the growth of bacteria, fungi and viruses.

- Tannins release antibacterial properties in the intestines and are also useful for burn treatment.

- Anthraquinone[11] are bitter compounds, and when used in high dosages, alleviate

---

[11] An excerpt from Wikipedia:

"Anthraquinone and Anthraquinone Derivatives are used as laxatives. The following plants and plant-parts constipation. Other effects documented by researchers are pain-relieving properties.

---

containing the anthraquinone substance are used in medicine: Senna (folia sennae) and its fruit, cascara rind (Rhamnus purshiana), rhubarb root (Rheum palmatum and Rheum officinale) and Aloe (Aloe capensis and Aloe barbadensis). They prevent the reabsorption of sodium through the intestinal lumen - in other words, anti-resorptive. Beyond that, this can trigger an inflow of liquids together with sodium, potassium, calcium and chloride-ions i.e. secretagogue. These effects lead to softer feces as well as an increased filling up of the colon. Through the stretching of the intestinal walls, the passing through the walls is accelerated and the defecation eased. The drug contains Anthraquinones as Glycosides. The sugars are separated from bacteria in the intestine, which is why the drug begins working here. The sugar-free Aglycones are also known as Emodins. They are reduced to Anthrones and Anthranols by the intestinal bacteria. These are the actual effective substances."

- Isoflavones reduce the increase of pathogens (germs) and are naturally anti-inflammatory.

The action spectrum of the above-mentioned bioflavonoid group, which can be broken down into further individual elements, is wide-ranging and broad.

Acemannan - the Immune System's Turbo Booster

The aloe contains a wide spectrum of important carbohydrates - such as aldopentose, galactose, glucuronic acid, glucose, mannose, rhamnose, xylose and celluloid.

One of the most important substances for our body is acemannan[12].

---

[12] Excerpt from Wikipedia:

"Acemannan has been demonstrated to induce macrophages to secrete interferon (INF), tumor necrosis factor-α (TNF-α) and interleukins (IL-1); therefore, it might help to prevent or abrogate viral infection. These three cytokines are known to cause inflammation, and interferon is released in response to viral infections. In vitro studies have shown acemannan to inhibit HIV replication; however, in vivo studies have been inconclusive.

Acemannan is currently being used for treatment and clinical management of fibrosarcoma in dogs and cats. Administration of acemannan has been shown to increase tumor necrosis and prolonged host survival; the animals have demonstrated lymphoid infiltration and encapsulation."

This substance is seen as a possible active ingredient in the fight against the HI-Virus and against certain types of cancer. Application and research in both areas is still on-going and can be seen as a possible treatment only. What has been determined by leading scientists, however, is acemannan's promotion of increased cellular respiration, which in turn, positively influences metabolism as well as aids detoxification of the body.

Other documented benefits include gastrointestinal cleansing, combined with an increase of healthy intestinal flora. This allows a facilitated breakdown of nutrients, which, in turn, eases and increases absorption through the intestinal walls.

Acemannan's effect of increased cell activity strengthens the body's natural defenses thereby further effectuating the body's defense mechanisms i.e. the antiparasitic, antiviral, antibacterial and antifungal properties are underlined. For this reason, aloe vera should always be a part of a bowel cleanse.

Vitamins - A Broad Spectrum of Beneficial Effects

Research has long established and proven that the presence of any one vitamin or vital substance is not the crucial factor, but a combination along with other substances. Many substances vital for our bodily functions can only be absorbed with the presence of other substances. Here, aloe vera is important as its 160 substances make for a wonderful combination with these vitamins and vital substances. The number of vitamins and their action spectrums are impressive and include the following:

- Vitamin A (Retinol) - positive effect on skin, eye sight, mucous membranes, respiratory passages and strengthening of the immune system

- Vitamin B1(Thiamin) strengthens the nervous system, muscles and cardiac function and is important for carbohydrate metabolism

- Vitamin B2 (Riboflavin) important for healthy skin, hair and nails, supports the digestive organs, has beneficial effects on the skin.

- Vitamin B6 (Pyridoxine) - has a positive effect on the nervous system and psyche (depression, mood swings, nervous conditions) and plays an important role in the protein metabolism (the digestion of proteins) as well as having a positive influence on your hormonal household and the immune system.

- Vitamin B12 (Cobalamin) - required for the development of red blood cells and positive effects for protein absorption. Vegans and vegetarians are often deficient in vitamin B12 as it is found mostly in meats. Aloe vera can be a wonderful ersatz.

- Folic Acid - important for cardio and circulation. It prevents high homocysteine[13]

---

[13] Wikipedia writes:

levels, which could lead to damage of the arteries and blood vessels. Pregnant women need increased amounts of folic acid to avoid premature births or miscarriages.

- Niacin - (used to be called Vitamin B3) supports metabolism and is needed to

---

"L-Homocysteine (Hcy) is a natural (non- proteinogenic) α-Aminosäure. It is a byproduct of the metabolism process during single carbon transfers. It occurs through S-Methylierung from L-Methionine as Methyl Donor. Increased blood levels of Homocysteine can damage the blood vessels and can result in increased blood levels of homocysteines. It is connected to depression and dementia in old age. Normal blood test lab results range between 5 and 10 $\mu mol \cdot l-1$. To regulate the homocysteine levels in the blood, a sufficient supply of betaine and Vitamins B12, B6 as well as folic acid is necessary. (...)"

build coenzymes. It strengthens the heart and is used to battle depression and disorders of the nervous system.

- Beta Carotene (aka Provitamin A) If needed, is converted into Vitamin A. Has a positive influence on eye sight and the immune system.

- Vitamin C (Ascorbic Acid) - supports wound-healing and strengthens the immune system. It is important for the regeneration of capillaries and blood vessels and strengthens the gums. A healthy supply of vitamin c prevents exhaustion and irritability.

- Vitamin E (aka Tocopherol) strengthen cell membranes and slows the aging process. Vitamin E plays an important role in lipometabolism and albumin metabolism. A healthy supply prevents nervous disorders and muscle weakness.

Minerals

Aloe vera offers a large diversity of vital minerals and trace elements. Here is a selection:

- Chloride - together with sodium, aids in the transmission of nerve impulses.

- Chromium - regulates lipometabolism and supports a whole row of enzymes. An adequate supply of chromium is crucial in the context of weight loss, as chromium is needed for the regulation of satiety

- Iron - is important for transporting oxygen throughout the bloodstream, supplying the cells. In turn, this has a crucial effect for the correct function, especially in regards to the immune system

- Potassium - regulates the water-electrolyte household. Together with calcium and chromium, potassium has positive effects on the muscles, in particular the heart.

- Copper - is important in avoiding rheumatic ailments.

- Magnesium - the anti-stress mineral. Is responsible for the smooth interaction between muscles and the nervous system. A magnesium deficiency can results in cramps and insomnia.

- Manganese - is important for the formation and activation of enzymes. Has influence in the production of insulin in the pancreas and increases the effect of Vitamin B1.

- Zinc - has a positive influence on the skin as well as on various hormones (for example the thyroid, growth and sexual hormones).

Amino Acids and Enzymes

Amino acids are protein building blocks. One differentiates between the essential (vital functions) and non-essential amino acids. The essential amino acids can not be produced by the body, are however, necessary for our body to be able to absorb proteins. We need twenty-two amino acids to do that (ten of which are essential amino acids)

Aloe vera provides twenty of the twenty-two amino acids and nine of the ten essentials.

Enzymes are proteins, acting as bio-catalysts, precipitating certain chemical reactions

These enzymes are in all body cells and have a significant influence on our metabolism as well as organ functions. Enzyme deficiencies can cause illnesses and metabolic diseases.

Aloe vera contains a broad palette of enzymes, playing a significant role in the detoxification process as well as lipometabolism functions.

Therapeutic Application of Aloe Vera

Statements and testimonies proclaiming aloe vera as a cure-all/wonder drug, able to heal and/or cure any sickness or illness, are simply incorrect and damages the reputation of this plant when used in reputable therapy. Therapists and healers do themselves and the promotion of the benefits and properties of aloe vera no favors when making such broad statements. It must be clearly understood that the ingestion of aloe vera gel, in whatever shape or form, will not counteract all negative influences (lifestyle/environment) we are exposed to.

Health and Vitality

Across many reports issued by users, medical professionals and healers, one finds the following beneficial applications:

- Allergic reactions through stings - Topical application of aloe vera gel.

- Gastrointestinal afflictions such as diarrhea, stomach cramps, constipation - Aloe vera gel in water offers relief. Ingestion of the gel soothes the intestinal walls, regulates digestion and is antifungal. Combining liquid ingestion with a bland diet is useful in this context.

- Eczema - Aloe vera gel is a well-tolerated alternative to antibiotics and cortisone products.

- Exhaustion - Aloe vera can mobilize reserves in the body and is also used in conjunction with burnout-syndrome. Naturally, a change of lifestyle must be considered as well.

- Colds, Flu - If you feel a cold coming on (runny nose, achy, etc), the ingestion of five to ten tablespoons of aloe vera gel daily, can stop the oncoming cold in its tracks.

- Joint pain - Aloe vera contains polysaccharides and amino sugars; these sugars have preventative and mitigating properties on joint functions. They support synovial fluid renewal. Aloe vera can be used topically (gel applied directly on the joints) or internally (ingestion of gel).

- Liver Maladies - Over a five-to-six-week period, drinking three to five glasses of water mixed with aloe vera gel aids the liver in its detoxification process. This cure is helpful when you've gone through a period of excessive alcohol consumption.

- Neurodermatitis - The cooling effect combined with the substances within aloe vera has been a popular treatment for patients suffering from this affliction and has done much to lessen the negative effects of this skin ailment.

- Psoriasis - So far, this skin ailment is not curable. However, the topical and internal use of aloe vera has been considered helpful in the battle against psoriasis. One additional benefit that has been established is that cell renewal is accelerated by the nutrients found in aloe vera.

- Sunburns - Applying aloe vera on the sunburnt skin is considered soothing. Here too, the nutrients in aloe vera - in topical applications - accelerate skin cell renewal, thereby mitigating the damaging effects of sunburn. Warning: sunburns can result in serious skin ailments such as melanoma. Melanoma and other pigmentation irregularities should immediately be checked by a medical professional.

There are many more symptoms that can be treated and/or alleviated with the use of aloe vera products. Many have been listed here and further usage of the plant and its products are introducing us to many more beneficial results going forward.

Consulting a medical professional regarding serious health issues should always be a priority. The beneficial substances in aloe vera have a lasting effect on strengthening the immune system, however, we do recommend any consumption to be discussed with your doctor or medical professional to determine the correlation between aloe vera and any other prescribed medication and/or ailment you may have.

Anti-Aging

The buzzword of our time: anti-aging. New products are flooding the market with increased regularity, all promising the same thing: youth. Unfortunately, the actual effects lag dramatically behind the marketing declarations most brands make.

As we know, the Egyptians called aloe vera ' the immortal plant.' However, it must be emphatically stated we cannot smooth away years of abuse (excessive food consumption, unhealthy food consumption, no exercise, etc) simply by using expensive skincare products. Having said that, aloe vera can be part of a successful strategy to battle the effects of premature aging and all that entails.

The anti-aging properties of aloe vera are being researched at the Health Science Center of the University of Texas. Aloe vera tested on animals has shown the beneficial properties in regards to health and life expectancy. Animals given a regular dose of aloe gel lived longer and were prone to fewer illnesses. How these findings will translate to humans has not been established as of yet.

Body Care

The unique substances found in aloe vera gel has been used for centuries in skincare, supplying nourishment and care for the body.

Skin loses its elasticity as we age. Our natural skin oils and moisture balance decreases as we grow older. Especially women notice these effects despite long term usage of various skin products (produced by the chemical industry). Despite spending massive amounts of money on skin care products, nothing seems to slow the aging process. The environment, air pollution, poor eating habits, stress, deficiencies, excessive UV exposure (or even worse, visits to the solarium) take a toll on our skin.

Aloe vera cannot reverse all these negative effects. However, if a serious effort is made, to reduce the negative factors in our lives that damage our health and especially our skin, aloe vera can be seen as a wonderful addition in achieving more positive results and effects for our health and our skin. Aloe vera cares for and maintains the natural beauty of our skin, improves the skin tone and elasticity, regulates its moisture household, and supports healthy skin if used over longer periods.

There are many cosmetic products available containing aloe vera. Many of these products contain a combination of aloe vera along with other beneficial substances. As is the case so often in life, the most expensive product is not always the best product. Pay attention to the ingredients; they should be natural products, and of high quality from organic sources, if possible. Also check the aloe vera gel percentage in the product.

DIY: Making Aloe Vera Gel and Aloe Vera Smoothies

To produce your own aloe vera gel, plants between the ages of three to five years are ideal (three-year-old plants from sunny regions; five-year-old plants from Central Europe). These are the ages where all the important ingredients have fully ripened.

To harvest aloe vera gel:

- cut a large aloe vera leaf from a living plant. Ideally, the leaf will be at least 20 cm long. We recommend not cutting leaves off the same plant too often so the plant does not lose its ability to regenerate, survive and prosper anew.

- Wash the leaf, place it upside down so the resin (the brown-green substance) can drain out. Resin has a diuretic effect i.e oral ingestion may cause diarrhea.

- There are two ways you can harvest the white gel: you either cut the leaf open and spoon out the gel or you can peel away the layers of the leaf. The former is advisable if you plan on using the gel side of the leaf as a mask for your skin.

The harvested gel can be eaten in small portions. It keeps well in sealed containers in the refrigerator for a few days. Do not freeze the gel!

You can also make smoothies. If you are new to aloe vera gel, use less than 10% of the harvested quantity, mix with water and (preferably organic) fruits and/or vegetables. Over time, you can increase the amount of aloe vera gel. Simply toss the portion of gel, water and the fruit (or vegetable) into you blender or mixer. Consume immediately. Store leftovers in your refrigerator - in a well-sealed container - for no more than a day.

At the outset of your journey with aloe vera gel, adults should not consume more than 1/10 liter of pure aloe-vera gel daily (or any other aloe vera gel product). It is important to note, that the correct dose is crucial to reaping the positive aspects and benefits of this amazing plant as overuse is potentially toxic with unpleasant side effects. We would like to stress that your medical professional may prescribe varying amounts during your aloe vera therapy.

Sources of Supply

Growing an aloe vera plant on your window sill is by far the most economical and cost effective way to have access to fresh aloe vera gel. But if you plan on consuming aloe vera gel on a daily basis, you will most likely not be able to meet your demand by growing your own plants. Luckily for us, there is a wide array of good aloe products available to buy.

Aloe vera gel, as well as its ingredients are sold in tablet or capsule form by many manufacturers. Prices vary from extremely high to extremely low.

Please consider the following before purchasing/deciding upon a particular product:

- Are the aloe plants from an organic source?

- How high is the actual aloe vera content? (some manufacturers dilute the aloe vera gel with over 90% useless fillers)

- Choose a product from a reputable source. Trusting no-name brands and low-cost manufacturers can hide health risks as some of the fill products used instead of high quality aloe vera gel can be dangerous to your health and well-being.

- Some manufacturers add sugar or artificial aromas to the aloe vera drinks. Again, we recommend reading the list of ingredients carefully before purchasing something you may not want to consume.

List of literature

- Barcroft, Alasdair: Aloe Vera: Nature's Silent Healer, 2003, Baam
- Bankhofer, Prof. Hademar: Aloe Vera - Die Pflanze für Gesundheit, Vitalität und Wohlbefinden, 2013, Kneipp Verlag, 6. Auflage
- Beringer, Alice: Aloe vera - Die Königin der Heilpflanzen: Natürlich gesund und schön durch den reinen Extrakt der Aloe vera, 2007, Heyne
- Delbé, Jean B.: Gesund werden - gesund bleiben: Aloe-Vera-Leitfaden Gesund bleiben, 2004, M+M Verlag
- Finnegan, John &, Schmid, Rainer: Aloe Vera - das Geschenk der Natur an uns alle, 2014, Ernährung & Gesundheit, 35. Auflage
- Oppermann, Jutta: Aloe Vera - Was die Pflanze wirklich kann, 2004, Lebensbaum
- Peuser, Michael: Kapillaren bestimmen unser Schicksal: Aloe - Kaiserin der

Heilpflanzen, Quelle für Vitalität und Gesundheit, 2010, St. Hubertus

- Rahn-Huber, Ulla: Natürlich heilen und pflegen mit Aloe Vera, 2015, Riwei
- Skinner, Rosalynd: Aloe Vera: The Medicine Plant, 2005, Mill Enterprises
- Skousen, Max B.: Aloe Vera Handbook: The Ancient Egyptian Medicine Plant, 2005, Book Publishing Company